CHILDREN DELIVERANCE

DELIVERANCE OF THE FOETUS

Spiritual Warfare in Pregnancy

Alexander Zabadino

Copyright © 2024 Alexander Zabadino

All rights reserved. No part of this book may be reproduced or transmitted in any form or by any means, electronic or mechanical, including photocopying, recording, or by any information storage and retrieval system without prior permission of the author.

This book is a work of non-fiction. The views expressed are solely those of the author and do not necessarily reflect the views of the publisher and thereby disclaims any responsibility for them.

This book is dedicated to God the Father, God the Son, and God the Holy Spirit

INTRODUCTION

This book interestingly uses a hybrid of proven spiritual and medical knowledge to give an understanding of how to nurture pregnancy, and deliver safely. It is well known that witchcraft can explore the star and destiny of an unborn child, and wage a spiritual war because of this, such that the baby is attacked, and maternal ignorance can be very expensive.

In polygamous settings of the world, and due to family issues, the wives could be envious of one another as to try to use spiritual means to investigate what the child is likely to become, as they attempt to bury the star of the child, or divert it. The operations of voodoo and other witchcraft technologies are no longer new.

Sometimes too, it may be a fault of the mother, through carelessness, or ignorance, which has been termed self-bewitchment in this book. In 1 Samuel 4:21, the daughter in law of Eli fell into panic, and her baby was attacked, and born prematurely, as a result of her emotions, even though the bible report says the time was near. This book mentions the various wicked acts that a foetus could be a victim of in the womb, and about 20 ways by which a foetus can be attacked in the womb, and the destiny perverted. This is why many children are born sick, deformed, disabled or spiritually incapacitated. Some of them only grow to be adults before they can discover the evil that has been done to them in the womb.

It is pertinent also for a mother to be able to know the various signs which point to a witchcraft attack of the foetus, and what each signifies. This may not be physical signs, but purely spiritual signs, which will only be noticeable in the dream. We have discussed thirty dreams that are relevant to deliverance of the foetus.

The bible makes us to know in James 4:3, that it is quite possible to pray, and receive not answers to prayers, because we did not pray the way we should, but have prayed based on our passions. The chapter on prayer strategies does not only give us the rationale based on which we should pray, but also outlines prayer points on the various problem areas.

Self-bewitchment is possible, if a mother is ignorant about certain things, and keep repeating the same mistakes over and over, especially the nutrition. This book examines in great detail, the various anomalies that could arise as a result of malnutrition, that is taking inappropriate diets during pregnancy, or a wrong balance between the nutrient types. For example, many mothers consume sea foods indiscriminately, not knowing that mercury in excess could cause developmental consequences in the new born.

The signs of labour and stages of labour have been highlighted especially for a first timer, in order to promote a sound understanding, and ensure a safe delivery. There are still certain things that women who have had babies once or twice may not understand. This book explains them in details that the mother will be able to follow with understanding, during labour.

An overview of the deliverance process is given at the end of the book for a clearer understanding of how to go about it, with a suggested timetable for the deliverance program.

Contents

CHAPTER 1 10
   WITCHCRAFT AGENDA FOR CHILDREN. 10

CHAPTER 2 16
   WICKEDNESS AGAINST THE FOETUS 16

CHAPTER 3 20
   20 ROUTES OF WITCHCRAFT ATTACK IN THE UNBORN CHILD. 20

CHAPTER 4 31
   SIGNS THAT THE BABY IS ATTACKED 31

CHAPTER 5 36
   DREAMS DURING PREGNANCY THAT REQUIRE YOUR ATTENTION. 36

CHAPTER 6 46
   PRAYER STRATEGIES FOR THE EXPECTANT MOTHER. 46

CHAPTER 7 76
   NUTRITION IN PREGNANCY 76

CHAPTER 8 82
   COMPLICATIONS IN PREGNANCY 82

CHAPTER 9 88
   FAITH IN PREGNANCY. 88

Chapter 10 98
   SIGNS OF LABOUR AND STAGES OF LABOUR. ...98
CHAPTER 11 107
   AN OVERVIEW OF THE DELIVERANCE OF THE FOETUS 107

This is to specially acknowledge the contributions of Miss. Elaine Choi Fung Chan for the typesetting and editing of this script, as well as designing a good cover for the book.

CHAPTER 1

WITCHCRAFT AGENDA FOR CHILDREN.

Children have been a target of the devil since the very time that Jesus was born! The wise men from the east saw his star, when it rose, and they came to worship him (Matthew 2:2). The glorious star and destiny of Jesus became a problem for King Herod. He sought to kill the baby Jesus, and was so desperate about this, that he killed many other children, born at that time in Jerusalem. The same is still the problem all over the world today, because there is always a Herod that is after every glorious child. It took the revelation of the three wise men, for Jesus to be delivered from the wickedness of Pharaoh. Till this time, the devil still keeps attacking children.

The truth is that in every household, every neighbourhood, and every organisation, there are people that have negative spiritual powers. With this, they could know which child carries a global glory, and would be a threat to their evil activities in the world, just like Herod. They therefore aggressively and viciously plan to destroy such children, thereby destroying what God has deposited in them, and the assignment given to them. If the parents are careless, or are not being guided by the highest power, then the enemy could easily have his way.

Some enemies attack children because they want to take revenge over them because of what their parents or grandparents did. As a result, these children are attacked in the womb. There are also some children that are suffering from an evil inheritance. The Bible says that our fathers have sinned and are not, but we have borne their iniquities (Lamentations 5:7), and if the foundations be destroyed, what can the righteous do? (Psalm 11:3).

There are some witchcraft powers, especially in the environment, that are after pregnant women, in order to attack the baby in their womb. They do this, because if they succeed, they receive more power in the kingdom of darkness. It could be likened in the opposite realm now, to a Pastor who wins the souls of children and does miracles. That goes on record of the ministry, and the Pastor will receive some recognition and accolades. It is so sad to note that the same happens in the kingdom of darkness, whenever parents are careless!

There are mothers who are into witchcraft covenant with witchcraft covens, familiar spirits, marine spirits, forest demons and all. When you have a covenant with demonic spirits, they are always with you, to supervise and perpetuate problems in your life, and in this case the life of the unborn baby. If the mother is possessed and the evil spirit is inside, and not just surrounding, people like that could bargain with the life of the child, their own lives, or both. Most still births happen like this, and doctors and midwives will try their bests, but still lose the child.

Curses could also be responsible, due to what the parents did and circumstances surrounding their marriage. Most broken marriage covenants at the time the parents were dating, often result to curses which fly and hit the unborn child. Psalm 74:20 says "have respect unto the covenant, for the dark places of the earth are full of the habitations of cruelty".

Sometimes, the attack on children in the womb is to cause a distraction to the career and marriage of the parents. There is no smarter move than to look for a way of attacking the unborn child. Unfortunately, immature parents blame one another for the outcome, instead of them to move closer and fight together, and have victory over the devil. They fight one another through their words and actions. Most times, the blame and all the care fall on the woman alone. Most careers especially of the women suffer, and the marriage could be turbulent, or broken.

There are several things that could be the result of witchcraft attacks in the womb. Usually, the plan of the devil is to steal, to kill and to destroy (John 10:10). There are so many negative tendencies observed in children, that could occur, if the parents were careless during pregnancy. This includes attack on the physical abilities of the child, and through witchcraft attacks, a child could be born lame, and a witch will confess, "we ate his legs, when he was in his mother's womb". The same witch would listen to the gospel, and get saved later.

I conducted deliverance for a teenager sometime around 2003. The demon inside her spoke, that "her grandmother handed her to us". She went further to say that "our assignment is to make sure that she doesn't have rest in life". This is why the poor girl was committing errors, and they will push her from one household to the other, as a house help, after committing one offence or the other.

Many children with cerebral palsy were attacked in the womb. All of a sudden, the spirit spouse will sleep with the mother in the dream, and spontaneously the mother would bleed, and lose blood. This blood loss affects the brain of the immature baby, giving rise to autism. There are several cases of women giving birth to children with animal features. Some children's head will be small and look like the head of a snake! In the hospital, they call it microcephaly, but it has a spiritual explanation. All these are destructive as well as stealing from the children.

Strange and deviant behaviour is another issue. Many children with unusual behaviour were attacked in their mother's womb. The bible says in Matthew 13:25, that while men slept, the enemy came, and sowed tares, and went his way. I pray that every tree not bearing fruit that was sown into the life of anyone, or any child while in their mother's womb shall be uprooted and cast into fire in Jesus name.

The truth is that the power to protect the children in the womb, or turn against evil inherited patterns, lies in the parents. There is so much that parents can do to prevent witchcraft attacks against the baby in the womb, and make them to be the best version that God has created them to be and wants them to be. There is quite a lot that mothers could do towards these, no matter how the enemy rages!

This book is basically for pregnant women, so that they can know their vulnerabilities and the extent to which the devil could go in order to attack babies. They will also learn how to prevent these terror attacks.

CHAPTER 2

WICKEDNESS AGAINST THE FOETUS

There are many casualties in many parts of the world, as the agenda of the devil is to pluck the star of every glorious child and make them useless, even from the womb. This is done in several ways, while the child is in the womb. If the parents are unable to help the child, and the child does not have an encounter with Jesus, it would be a great disaster as children like that may die sorrowful, wasted, and unfulfilled. That was why Jesus came to set the captives free.

The way the witches attack is somehow complex, because after the attacks, there will always be a medical explanation for some. Some of these things will happen, but there is no explanation for it. A pregnant mother could dream that someone actually came to her in the dream, in the early hours of the day, at dawn, to press her Tommy. Afterwards, she started having pain, and bleeding.

The result could be a brain damage on the child. The doctors can diagnose cerebral palsy, but the process that leads to that was complex.

Many children with promising destinies have been robbed like that while their mothers were pregnant, only for someone to confess openly in the market place, that in our coven, we ate the brain. They may also go further to tell you close relatives of the parents that participated in the evil act. Such a child would have problems academically. If the parents do not understand spiritual things, but believe just on medical reports alone, then they wouldn't pray or fast about it. They just resign to fate and the child carries the problem for life.

A child may be made blind in the womb, or deaf, because a strange personality appeared to the mother in the dream and injected her. Dreams of injections of the pregnant mother in the dream should not be taken with levity. The blood becomes infected and may lead to infections of the affected organs.

A wicked spirit from an altar in the environment could jump into the baby inside especially if a pregnant mum likes to go out late at night, or too early in the morning. Some people do rituals in the night or early hours of the morning. Someone passes by, and all of a sudden feel goose bumps all over the body, that is an evil spirit. There are people that bathe of drop other fetishism materials at the road junction.

Strange behaviours in children are another problem. There are children that will never obey simple instructions, both at home, and at school, or anywhere. These children face rejection in their lives because of these behaviours. It makes it difficult for them to succeed in anything they do. In this type of manipulation too, evil spirits might enter into the womb.

The truth is that some of these demons do not manifest immediately, but keep growing until a later date. There are mothers that are the manhood of their children, when they were in the womb. They shared it to their sacred mates. The child may not see it as a serious issue, until he is married and is expecting to be a father. Many parents harvest the organs of their unborn babies, diabolically in the womb in exchange for favours, material or spiritual.

There have been reported cases in the past of women that gave birth to animals like snakes, cats, or dogs. There was a reported case of someone who gave birth to a stone. All these are witchcraft manipulations. Sometimes the babies are half human and half animal. Conjoined twins do have a medical explanation, but are the works of the witchcraft.

There are also die-hard habits that were programmed in the womb. When these die-hard habits manifest, people are of the opinion that it happened since the time they were in the womb and old enough to be changed. However, this idea is a lie! There is no one that Jesus cannot change and whenever there is a will, there is a way.

The developmental stages of a baby's life happen in the womb. The enemy seeks to arrest this development. Nearly all the children with one form of disability or the other were born with it, meaning they were attacked in the womb.

CHAPTER 3

20 ROUTES OF WITCHCRAFT ATTACK IN THE UNBORN CHILD.

There are routes of witchcraft attack in the unborn child, which could be explored by witchcraft. Majority of these routes are opened to witchcraft attacks because of the fault on the part of the mother. The following 20 channels are prominent.

Food. Food bought on the high street are more prone to be used by witches for attacking the unborn baby. The ingredients used in cooking, the people that cooked, where they cooked, the method of cooking, and the likes, if not verified pose potential dangers spiritually against the child, especially if you are known to be a regular customer. For example, if they know that you come to buy breakfast every morning. They could pre-pack bewitched food for you, so that you eat it with problems arising.

It is also possible to bewitch yourself through food as a pregnant woman. The nurses would always tell you that excessive carbohydrates are not good for the weight of the baby. If the baby has excessive weight, you might be operated upon. The food substances, proteins, fats and oils, minerals and vitamins have to be taken in the right portions, otherwise health problems arise and you would have bewitched yourself.

Spirit husband. A spirit husband is a personality that often appears in the dream to have sex with the pregnant woman. The agenda of the spirit husband is to spiritually violate the pregnant woman, causing harm to the baby, or introducing toxins into the system, in order to cause infections or similar problems. Women that have lust towards other women's husband or actually have sex with them are open to the attack of spirit husbands. Dressing with artificial attachments are also prone to attacks of spirit husband as well as people that engage in dirty discussions and other obscene acts.

Consultation with the mediums. A pregnant woman who is expectant should not go to palmists, necromancers, or star gazers for consultation. Each time you do this, you expose yourself and your baby to evil spirits. The palmistry is not doing all that with their powers, but they have evil personalities that are behind their activities. These powers can leap inside the baby and commit evil. Mothers should desist from going to palmistry and star gazers.

Concoctions. Concoctions are magical preparation aimed at healing or solving some spiritual problems in native and unconventional means. The ingredients are products of leaves and animals that work mystically, most of the time. Usually, spirits are summoned during the preparation of these concoctions which appear wherever the concoctions are being used. The devil does, unlike God, does not have a free gift, but he operates a trade-by-barter system. He could take away back pain during pregnancy and give you an autistic child. This is why it is dangerous to drink concoctions. The power source is questionable and this could lead to problems later in life.

Idol festivals. There are festivals celebrated to honour idols. During the celebration of these festivals, there are other idol priests that attend the occasion, thereby building up a heavy traffic of demons and numerous invisible and negative spiritual transactions. A pregnant woman who attends this type of gathering, stands a risk of the transfer of demons, not just in the atmosphere, but through eating and drinking. Weird dances are body movements, as well the eye gate transfer demons. What you see will leave a lasting impression, and attending such gatherings is unsafe for a pregnant woman.

Maternal demonic possession. When a pregnant woman is possessed by a demon, then she is totally under the control of the demon that has possessed her, such that she makes spiritual decisions and transactions, that do not fall under their consciousness and control. Some women confess that they were responsible for the death of their babies, or disability in their babies. Some of them made terrible agreements against the welfare of their babies. Others made a covenant to die on the day of delivery in the labour room.

Evil covenants of parents. Apart from being possessed by a demon, there are parents who entered in covenants with different sects or objects, which impact negatively upon the wellbeing of their unborn babies. This may be a covenant with the occult for people seeking to be wealthy. Some of them make covenants with trees, rivers or mountains. There are cults that specifically request for the blood of a pregnant woman, and sometimes it has to be the blood of someone that they love so much, or their pregnant wife. This is generally called blood money.

Prayerlessness. There is no condition that prayer cannot turn around, in as much as we care to ask God. He says in Jeremiah 33:3 that "call unto me in the day of trouble, and I will answer thee, and do great and mighty things which thou knowest not." A lazy Christian has immense potentials and ability to receive favours from God. However, many do not pray, thereby they cannot receive great things or protection from God. A pregnant woman could also simply pray for angelic assistance for protection or other benefits. If they don't pray, then they lose out of these things.

Incisions. Razor or knife cuts on the skin, with the rubbing of magical powders into these cuts are common in many traditions, which believe that they are medicinal and protective. However, in actual fact, they pollute the blood spiritually. Many kinds of fetishism materials like the eyes of a wall gecko, teeth of a snake, skin of animals, and many strange magical ingredients are ground into powder and rubbed directly into the blood. This opens the door for demons and diverse types of spiritual attacks in the dream which affect the unborn baby negatively. These may affect the physical development of the baby giving rise to congenital malformations or brain retardation.

Attacks from environmental altars. Most environments that pregnant women find themselves are not friendly in the least. There are different possessed human beings, possessed animals, and trees and rivers for example that are possessed by demons. There is no way that a pregnant woman can totally avoid interaction with these parties. These hibernating demons in the environment can see the glory of unborn babies and are ready to steal, kill or destroy, but resting on God's power, this shall be impossible.

Abuse of medication and drugs. This is more or less self bewitchment by choice or disobedience. There are a list of medications and chemical substances that must not be taken by pregnant women. This is why you need to check from the literature or pamphlet inside any pack of medication, if it is safe for you to use. The wrong medications have negative effects on the growth and development of unborn babies, like making them to have excess digits, blindness, disability etc. Non-Steroidal Anti-Inflammatory drugs (NSAIDS) which include ibuprofen, diclofenac, aspirin, are normally pain relief or anti-inflammatory drugs, but could cause heart problems in babies or reduces the amniotic fluid, which protects the foetus from injury and temperature changes. The use of tetracycline is normally as an antibacterial, but it could cause inhibited bone growth in babies, as well as teeth discolouration. Drinking of alcohol in pregnant mothers can cause growth retardation, facial anomalies, and central nervous system dysfunction. Tobacco causes low birth weight, premature birth, and increased risk of sudden infant death syndrome (SIDS).

Eating in the dream. When a person is greedy and gluttonous, eating everything, or eating at the wrong hours, there are demons that observe this and leverage on this anomaly to feed a pregnant woman with rubbish and potentially dangerous substances in the dream. This can make a pregnant woman to be sick and unwell, during and after pregnancy. Food in the dream also affects the physical and spiritual well-being of the unborn baby.

Laying of hands. One major way of transferring positive or negative spiritual powers is by laying of hands. Under no condition, should a pregnant woman allow anyone to lay hands on any part of their body. Many people transfer negative power in that manner. This negative power can accomplish whatever they have sent them to accomplish. A man once confessed that he wiped off the star of an unborn baby, while he was in the womb. The child grew up to be vagabond and several times was homeless. This could have been prevented if the mother could say no to touching or laying of hands.

Exposure to rays. There are two major types of rays that are potentially dangerous. The first is the ionising radiation, which includes x-rays, and gamma rays. The second and less harmful rays is the non-ionizing radiation which includes waves from smartphones, and electro-magnetic waves from electronic equipment.

Satanic gifts during wedding. The wedding time is the time that the enemy rages through gifts. There are satanic gifts sometimes that are dedicated or cursed.

When a person receives such a gift, it affects the baby or the mother. The negative possibilities are endless, if a person receives a satanic gift.

Eye gaze attacks. There are witches that have power in the eyes. They only need to fix their gaze on the belly of the pregnant woman, and make a wish. I pray that every evil desire of witchcraft, over you or your baby shall backfire in the name of Jesus Christ. As they fix the gaze, evil anointing is transferred into the life of the baby or the mother. This could have a negative effect on the life of the baby.

Indifference to dreams. Dreams are established by God to give us information or instructions that are helpful in delivering us from the bondage of the evil one. Dreams are extremely important and we need to be serious with dreams, interpreting them to know the meanings, and acting upon each meaning for solution to problems. Every pregnant woman should have a dream book/journal to keep records of events in their lives, and refer when needed.

Demonic possession in the father. If the father of the unborn baby has any evil traits or possession, it could be transferred through blood. A demonic possession in the life of the father will also cause negative things in the life of the unborn baby. This is why the children can inherit problems from the life of the father, and it starts from right inside the womb.

Curses in the life of the parents. Parents may have done something wrong or bad and as a result, God curses them, or they are cursed by man as of a result of their evil deeds. The children may be part of the sufferers of what the parents did. In 2 Kings 5:27, Gehazzi was cursed, and his seed forever. Elisha said "now the leprosy of Naaman shall cling unto thee and unto thy seed forever." The children of Gehazzi automatically were carriers of leprosy in the womb, as a result of being cursed.

Astral projections. In astral projection, a person separates the astral body or spirit from the physical body, and does an out of body experience (OBE) to a different location that they want, to interact with spiritual beings in the spirit world and have an impact upon their lives. Witches do it to the unborn baby in order to do evil. However, if you allow the power of the Holy spirit to fill you and you are prayerful, a nasty experience like that can't happen.

Blood suckers and flesh eaters. One of the greatest attackers in the spirit world, of pregnant women, are the blood suckers and flesh eaters. They are the ones responsible, when people have motor traffic accident, and lose blood. They are the ones responsible, when people menstruate and loose a lot of blood. They are also the ones responsible, when people are putting to bed, they are losing blood and the blood cannot be stopped. They are also the ones responsible when a pregnant woman, all of a sudden sees herself in a pool of blood, thereby having an abortion or almost having an abortion. When a pregnant woman loses a lot of blood, it affects the baby, and the baby may not be born healthy.

Careless with underwear. Witchcraft attacks due to careless exposure of underwear are common! The wicked ones can take panties, bras, and other underwear to the kingdom of darkness to wreak havoc on the woman and on the baby. The blood sucking witches also use underwear to achieve their bad goals. Flesh eaters are responsible for sick organs, for example, a child born with a swollen eye, or other parts of the body abnormally sick.

CHAPTER 4

SIGNS THAT THE BABY IS ATTACKED

It is a common thing for babies to be attacked in the womb, because the mother is not sensitive. The various signs include:

Bleeding through the vagina. This is one of the most common signs that show that an unborn baby may be attacked. Bleeding through the vagina most likely reveals a miscarriage, ectopic pregnancy, placental abruptness in which case the placenta separates from the uterus preterm labour, uterine rupture. All cases of bleeding through the vagina should be reported without delay to your doctor. However, the truth is that if a mother is prayerful enough, things like this would have been revealed and appropriate steps taken.

Bad dreams. The dreams that we have is a spiritual picture of what is happening to us. The Bible says in Job 33:15 "in a dream, in a vision of the night, when deep sleep falleth upon men, in slumberings upon the bed; then he openeth the ears of men and sealeth their instruction, that he may withdraw man from his purpose, and hide pride from man. He keepeth back his soul from the pit, and his life from perishing by the sword." Just as "the spirit of man is the candle of the Lord" (Proverbs 20:27). Whenever there is a violation of God's commandments, demonic forces move in to attack. Every plan of the enemy by you can be revealed to you, so that you can avert them. Thank you, Jesus. There are many types of dreams that a pregnant woman can have, which carry different meanings. Dreams in pregnancy and their interpretations will be discussed in another chapter, later in this book.

Sickness. Sudden illness during pregnancy is not a good sign, and also should be taken care of. It is possible to eat, drink, or be injected in the dream, with sudden illness the following day or next. A high fever will normally indicate a generalised infection in the mother, which may affect the child, especially the brain, which is not yet mature, or the respiratory system. Cases like that could lead to permanent brain damage or to the lungs which are not well developed too.

Reduced foetal movement. A person may have sex during pregnancy and wake up to discover that there is very little or no foetal movement in the womb. This indicates that something is wrong, or the baby is dead in the womb, and should be reported to the doctor immediately. Evil people could also project into the baby in an astral projection and cause havoc. Intra uterine death calls for urgent attention so that the baby does not decompose inside the mother and cause sepsis.

Constant fear. 2 Timothy 1:7 says, "for God has not given us a spirit of fear, but of power, and of love, and of a sound mind." This clearly shows that fear is not of God. Fear is a sign that something has gone wrong, which most times is there but cannot be pinpointed objectively. In times like this, we need prayer and the study of the word. Usually after praying, you catch a revelation which takes fear away and gives boldness. Anytime you have a witchcraft attack, you tend to be afraid, or when an organ is dysfunctional. Counsel is the first line of action.

Hearing strange voices. Some voices may say frightening things into your ears, during pregnancy, like we shall kill you, or we make you suffer or other strange things. This makes most women, to be afraid, especially people who are getting own pregnant for the first time.

Visions that frighten. If the witchcraft powers have linked up with you through food, or sex, they can bring false visions that frighten. A mother in law may link you through blood (of her son), and attack you from there. If you get intimidated and devastated, then she can use that too.

Feelings as if someone is following you, or with you in the room. This often signifies the presence of an evil monitor, or demonic twin sister.

Severe abdominal pain. Severe abdominal pain could be the first signal of a witchcraft attack, then followed by blood. Severe abdominal pain during pregnancy may indicate ectopic pregnancy, pre-term labour, placental abruption (separation of the placenta from the uterine wall) or uterine rupture.

Severe headache and high blood pressure. These could be as a result of pre-eclampsia in a pregnant woman. This presents with high blood pressure, and protein in the pee. They are often picked up during antenatal appointments. It is an emergency as the blood pressure needs to be controlled. The patient may be detained in the hospital. Signs of pre-eclampsia include severe headache, vision problems, pain below the ribs, vomiting and sudden swelling of the hands, face and feet, shortness of breath, and decreased urination. In severe pre-eclampsia, it may involve the kidneys and the liver.

Visual changes. This is usually associated with blurring and flashing. However, pregnant women retain a lot of fluid, resulting in changes in thickness and shape of the cornea, and causing a distorted vision. This would usually be reversed after delivery or after breastfeeding.

Severe swelling. Some degree of swelling is normal in a pregnant woman, but should not be obscene and alarming. Swelling may increase in the lower extremities especially in hot weather, and after standing for a long time. The pressure occasioned by the weight of the baby could also obstruct the venous return. Pre-eclampsia causes swelling of the ankles and feet.

Fluid leakage from the vagina before 37 weeks. This is an abnormal case in which the membranes in the womb protecting the baby are broken, and that could open up the baby to infection and sepsis. It could also lead to pre-term labour.

CHAPTER 5

DREAMS DURING PREGNANCY THAT REQUIRE YOUR ATTENTION.

Sex in the dream. Sex in the dream is an attack of spirit husband. The mission of the spirit husband is to abort your pregnancy or make your unborn baby challenged physically or mentally. Try not to indulge in rough play with people you are not married to. Also, if you are not properly married, the devil may wage war through spirit husband. He sees it as not right for you to have a child for whosoever you are not legally married to. Furthermore, make sure you dress appropriately. Many pregnant women dress loosely, and this attracts spirit husband and makes him to attack you. Pray for mercy, which rejoiceth against judgement, and the Lord to deliver you.

Having children in the dream when you are pregnant. If you have spirit husband, definitely, you are most likely to have spirit children. The thing here is that the spirit children will appear in your dreams to attack your pregnancy. It is possible to see them fight you or attack the baby in the womb, or do other things against your baby. Then you need to bind them, and release the fire of God upon them. Withdraw their power and strength in the name of Jesus Christ.

Eating in the dream. When you are pregnant, you need to strictly control your eating habits. If your eating habits are rough, that is eat anywhere, any food cooked by any one, at anytime, anywhere, then you are a good candidate that the enemy will like to feed in the dream.

Naming ceremony in the dream. Naming ceremony in the dream as a pregnant woman is not good, and is a reverse dream. Most times, the naming ceremony or wedding that has been done in the dream cancels the right to do it physically. You need to pray seriously against sorrow and every evil. Know that there is nothing that God's power can't do.

Dreams of pepper, tomatoes, palm oil, all very ripe and red, has to do with blood. You need to check yourself to make sure you avoid any bleeding by injury or otherwise. It may also translate to anaemia in the unborn, which is common. Then when you have dreams like this, as you pray, you work on your nutrition. Eat well to nourish your baby.

Anomalies about the baby in the womb. Sometimes, by inheritance or spiritual transfer or exchange, you may discover strange things about the baby in the womb, like dreaming that your baby is an adult, or painted chalk on the face, or some other strange things. Never mind, just lay your hands on the tummy and begin to release fire on the baby. Anoint your tummy, and drink a lot of anointing oil. Pray purging prayers which you will see in my earlier book "Complete Deliverance from Witchcraft".

Pressing the baby in the womb. It is sometimes possible for a pregnant woman to be pressed by known or unknown persons in the dream. This is a sign that there are evil powers that are after your baby to do him or her evil. If you have any issues, or have offended anyone, then ask for mercy. Put the mark of the Lord Jesus on your baby, and decree that let no power trouble your baby any longer.

Injection in the dream, or medication in the dream. When a nurse or doctor injects you in the dream, or they give you medication to take, it is not a good dream. It is a means of introducing toxins into your system and that of your baby, to make you sick or do some other harm. Then you need to neutralise them with the blood of Jesus, and arrest their evil activities.

Bleeding in the dream. Leviticus 17:11 says, "the life of the flesh is in the blood." Anytime you lose blood in the dream; life and vitality is being taken away from you in a scenario that it translates to sickness. Actually, losing blood in the dream drains life out of you or your baby and points to a possible sickness. Then you pray to receive strength, and pray disease prevention prayers.

Sickness in the dream. When a person is sick in the dream, it means the spirit of infirmity is attacking. The type of infirmity may be similar to that which you have seen in the dream, for example, a swollen neck in the dream could also mean a swollen neck in waking life. When you have a dream, then you pray to hear from God, and take some actions.

Dead people, coffins, cemetery, owls all signify the spirit of death. God wants to deliver from the spirit of death (Job 33:17), and that is why you are seeing this. The dead people you see may be dead relatives, or members of your family. The fear of death may grip you, but you need to pray against it and ignore it. Some ladies start fearing death at child birth at a very young age, even though it is not the plan of God for them. Hallelujah.

Cows with horns, black birds, snakes, lions, crocodiles and every wild animal you see in the dream indicate that you have witchcraft contending against you, and you need to fight spiritual warfare. Sometimes, the animals may just be from the riverine environment, and you know you are fighting a battle against marine personalities. Marine personalities are the ones that sponsor spirit spouse, and spirit children, most commonly.

Evil summons by witches is common. In the dream, all of a sudden, you see yourself in a room, surrounded by people. They ask you questions and they try to judge you. They may decide to pass any judgement. The Bible says that mercy rejoiceth against judgement. There is nothing that they can do to overpower you if you have Jesus Christ and believe his power. Another thing is to always try as much as possible to be blameless.

Dreams about former boyfriend. If you have been in a relationship with anyone, and there are issues between both of you that implicate you, the devil can bring it to challenge you. If you promised to marry him for example, and you didn't eventually, he could appear in the dream and starts cursing you. I pray that iron-like curses shall not prosper in your life in the name of Jesus Christ. A woman had a vow with a boyfriend that she was going to marry him. The boy died in an accident but the woman continued to see him because the covenant was not broken. If she was pregnant, the boy could have killed the baby or done something harmful.

Pursued in the dream. This means that some enemies are after you, or that you have issues to settle with them. If you offended anyone, then ask for forgiveness. If these people make any statement in your dream, as they pursue you, then note it. What actually are they trying to do? Are they trying to kill you, or are they trying to collect something from you? What was the outcome of the dream? Did they catch up with you or not? What colour of dress were they putting on- red, or black, or multi-colour. What did you tell them in the dream?

Marine or water dreams. It is not uncommon to have water dreams during pregnancy, if you have spirit spouse. The spirit spouse will like to attack your fertility, and for this reason, you may see a spirit spouse making love to you, or trying to fight you. If this is the case, then you need to pray covenant breaking prayers in my book "Complete Deliverance from Witchcraft". Breaking of covenants in pregnancy is very good. We shall see how to pray during pregnancy, shortly. Dreams about swimming in the water that you had in the past or now are relevant, and should be addressed.

Dreams about people pressing you in the dream. Any dream about people pressing you in the dream, needs to be urgently discussed with your Pastor, or you could contact me. Any other rough or wicked acts should be addressed. This certainly shows that they are after your baby, and you should not just keep quiet and not pray. Join prayer programs for pregnant women.

Strange voices. Strange voices could be heard in the dream, or ordinarily when you are resting. It may also come as something you are feeling. It is as though you are hearing something like that inside you. These voices usually do not say good things concerning you, and tend to frighten you. Don't worry anyways! The devil always likes to harass and intimidate you, so that you are afraid and fall for his threats. However, if you pray and confess God's word continuously and violently, he loses his power. Do not give the devil the chance to intimidate you, and ride over you.

Barriers. Anything that will not allow you to move ahead in a dream is a barrier. There are spiritual barriers, which you must address. Imaginations, thoughts, doubts, unbelief, emotions and feelings are all barriers that you need to overcome in your pregnancy. Anytime you see a wall or barrier in your dream, it points to any or a combination of these factors.

Lonely dreams. Some people have lonely dreams depending on their context. It might be a dream of feeling lonely at home, at work, or on the day of your delivery. A pregnant woman may dream that they are alone on the day of their delivery, which happens to some women. When the time to put to bed is near, the husband and family of a pregnant woman should make sure that they give her the necessary support, and be there to help if she suddenly falls into labour.

Dreams about thick darkness. This is suggestive of a situation of ignorance and uncertainty. Anyone having this type of dream have certain things she does not know. Secondly, wicked people may surround her at the moment, and she needs to pray for the light of God to fall upon her life, and illuminate her darkness. Sometimes, you might need to pray for God to reveal secret things to you, as you read secular books for more knowledge and understanding.

Similitudes, or symbolisms. There are symbols that you see, or similitudes that you see, which tell you a lot about what happened in the past to you, or things that will happen. For example, you may dream to see a goat, delivering easily. The similitude is referring to you. Also, you may see a goat giving birth to twins. That is referring to you.

Names of people. Dreaming to see people you saw last many years back, might not really make sense to you. However, you see that people with you in a dream are Joy, Mercy, Blessings, which means that all these things are your portion, and will soon happen to you. The names of the people that you see in your dreams, especially if for a long time carries meanings. The meaning of those names in your local dialect too is relevant.

Dreams about the hospital. If you pray every day to God, to show you secrets about the hospital where you registered for ante-natal care, and you want to deliver there, God will show you secrets you need to know about the hospital. If the hospital is not good enough, God will show you something strange about it in your dream. If any of the staff is not clean, God will show you, and the way the dream will show you, it will be obvious to you, the next steps that you need to take.

Utterances in the dream. Be mindful of any utterances in the dream that you made or that any other person made concerning you or your situation. The utterances matter a lot and usually reveal the truth of what is happening. However, the one that is not favourable, you can change it through your prayers and your actions.

CHAPTER 6

PRAYER STRATEGIES FOR THE EXPECTANT MOTHER.

Prayer (communication) with God is important as a pregnant woman, to confess your faults to God, to ask for God's mercy, to seek God's face concerning certain things you would like God to do for you. God likes speaking with man, and keeps repeating his words for understanding, but unfortunately, we do not perceive (Job 33:14)

A pregnant woman who is going to work and is not that heavy (especially in the first and second trimesters of pregnancy) should be able to pray up to two times daily, in the morning, and in the evening.

The prayers should be structured, depending on certain needs and lifestyle of the expectant mother. A pregnant woman is not expected to fast or abstain from food beyond 12 noon, on Aby day they want to fast. A good and balanced nutrition is essential for excellent maternal health and foetal development.

What are the things to consider in prayer?

Forgiveness of sins. The Bible makes us to know that "for all have sinned and come short of the glory of God" (Romans 3:23). If we say we have no sin, we lie, and the truth is not in us (1 John 1:8). Every sin we have committed must be confessed before God, and we ask for forgiveness. The enemy is looking for unconfessed sins that he wants to use as a stronghold to attack you. The bible says that as many as confess their sins and forsake them shall obtain mercy (Proverbs 28:13).

Mercy of God. After asking for forgiveness from God, the next thing is to ask for the mercy of God. Mercy cancels judgement (James 2:13), and rolls away punishment. If you have done anything wrong to anyone in the past, you should ask for the mercy of God, and he will pardon. This is to avoid unfortunate circumstances. It is one of the secrets of warfare - mercy!

Break covenants. There are several unconscious covenants, that we keep entering into daily. This may be through food, through sex, through careless words of mouth, through where we went to and so on. These covenants have joined us to people places or things, and we keep seeing them in our dreams. These covenants need to be prayed against aggressively, and broken. Then we can be free from some problems, some of which are relevant in pregnancy and childbirth.

Curses. This is a force or influence, that works contrary to people's expectations and ambitions. Sometimes, it could be spoken against someone, and sometimes merely by an act of omission (something we ought to have done, but didn't do) or a commission (something we ought not to have done, but we did). For example, if we refuse to show kindness to others, but we don't, a curse is in place, because we can't receive kindness. Anything that the bible prescribes must be done in obedience.

Evil dedication. Some people through the direct worship of idols, or through idol worship by their ancestors, were joined to idols, and dedicated. Their lives will be under control by these demons, and certain sicknesses, known in the hospital as "hereditary" were acquired through that means. Unfortunately, many pregnant women fall under this category, having one disease or the other. Some miscarry spontaneously for no clear medical reason, but Behold, such phenomenon has spiritual explanations. The yoke of evil dedication is responsible for many problems, but good enough, they can be broken.

Divine provision. A pregnant woman needs to pray for divine provision for her family, in addition to whichever the husband must have prayed. Money is needed for the hospital bills, consumables, entertainment of guests, and many others. An expectant family should endeavour to save towards financial security, from the first month of pregnancy. They should pray for opportunities that will bring financial breakthroughs, as well as helpers and favours.

Hospital divinely prepared. It is not just enough to choose a hospital, because some of the hospitals are just glossy, but don't have good staff, and some don't have a good system put in place. It is more or less like a trap, and if you are in such a trap, then you need to pray yourself out of it. God may often show you the name of the hospital, or make you to hear it, sometimes not just in your dream, but you may just sit down and your mind would wander to the hospital, and as you think of it, you have peace!

Good staff. Pray that God should link you up with good staff, that he will use to favour you. Pray that he should give you the right attitude to find the favour of good staff. Sometimes, it also depends on your character, and not just the staff. It means you need to be calm, obedient and well behaved to the people that you meet. Everything is not just about our prayers, but also our behaviour and attitude, such that even when you have prayed, your attitude, and behaviour could hinder your prayers.

Divine wisdom. There is nothing that can be compared to the wisdom of God, because it is infallible and perfect. We need to pray for the staff, that God should give them every wisdom that they need to assist us and for us to give glory to God at the end of everything. We also need wisdom to navigate and to interact with people. This borders on our ability to be able to do God's will per time. Everything you want to do, comes two voices, the "do it" or "don't do it". Try to sincerely identify that which aligns with God's word, and follow it. It will always give you peace.

Bind and loose! Learn to pray the prayers of binding. Every being, responsible for every negative action should be bound in the name of Jesus. Focus as you repeatedly bind them. Everything that is good that you want, should loose from where they are bound in the name of Jesus. You should also loose yourself, your spirit from every evil altar in the name of Jesus.

Blood of Jesus. Jesus shed his blood on the cross of Calvary for the remission of sins. We were justified by the blood of Jesus and adopted as sons. The blood of Jesus carries a cleansing power that we need to use the blood of Jesus against demons. Whenever we pray, especially against demons, the blood of Jesus is so potent. It is also great to drink the blood of Jesus. Just continue saying, I drink the blood of Jesus Christ for up to 45 minutes or 60 minutes. Also sing songs like "there is power mighty in the blood". Always soak your baby in the blood of Jesus Christ.

Protection over you and your family. Pray generally for protection over every member of your family. Call upon the fire of the Holy Ghost to incubate them as well. Pray that they shall not harbour bewitchment for you and your baby.

Anointing oil. Try and get a bottle of anointing oil and bottled water, and make sure that you have it at home all the time. Pray into the oil and water, that finger of God, stir my oil/water. This oil/water, turn into the blood of Jesus Christ. Fire of the Holy Ghost, incubate my oil/water. You my oil/water, carry the miracle power of God, and begin to work signs and wonders in the name of Jesus Christ. Power of Protection from the throne of grace, enter into my oil/water in the name of Jesus Christ. Power that knows no impossibility, enter into my oil/water in the name of Jesus Christ.

Holy Spirit. The Holy Spirit is our senior partner, and is everywhere, knows everything and can do all things. If you are already baptised in the Holy Ghost, then you need to strengthen your spirit every morning, and at all times as you speak in the Holy Ghost. This protects your baby too, and impacts the Holy Ghost into the spirit of the child. If you fellowship with the Holy spirit, he will reveal many things to you, and always give you strength. Build the wall of fire around your baby in the name of Jesus Christ.

Incubate your child. Always incubate your child in the fire of the Holy Ghost. Lay your hands on your womb and continuously pray, "fire of the Holy Ghost, incubate my baby", and protect my baby in the name of Jesus Christ. You my baby, receive strength, you are a Victor, you are not a victim.

Destroy every environmental evil altar. An altar is a place of exchange, between a deity and a subject. There are people and powers that operate on altars and bring problems to the community. Sometimes the pandemics like cholera, measles, meningitis and the likes. As you destroy the altars, you bind the powers operating upon them too. There are altars in the waters, known as marine altars, altars in the graveyard, on trees, in the heavenlies all pertinent to your environment.

Frustrate the token of the wicked. There are weapons of spiritual warfare, with which you can frustrate the token of the wicked. Brimstone of fire, earthquake of God, liquid fire of God, anger of God, blood of Jesus, fire of the Holy Ghost.

Break the power of blood suckers. Blood sucking demons are interested in attacking pregnant women, and their attacks cause tremendous loss of blood, suddenly during pregnancy or at the time of labour and delivery. Haemorrhage is one of the most dreaded complications of pregnancy, and you need to bind blood suckers, and prohibit them spiritually from coming near your dwelling.

Prayers for forgiveness and mercy.

Father, forgive me for every sin of negative pronouncements over my life and my destiny.

I ask for the forgiveness of the sins of my ancestors, that wants to work against me on the day of my delivery.

Every sin, that wants to chase away my helpers in my pregnancy, and on the day of my delivery, O Lord, take it away from me.

Mercy that rejoiceth against judgement, prevail over my situation in the name of Jesus Christ.

Do some almsgiving periodically, like every Thursday, and say, mercy of God, overshadow my life, throughout the day, and ask God for what you want.

Every sin against my ex-boyfriend that is crying against my safe delivery, I wipe you away by the power in the blood of Jesus

I ask for forgiveness for every sin of abortion in the past, in the name of Jesus Christ.

Every evil handwriting upon my life, as a result of my sin, be blotted out by the power in the blood of Jesus Christ.

Evil altars, sponsoring iniquity in my life, be destroyed by the fire of the Holy Ghost.

I overcome every condemnation in my life as a result of sin, by the power in the blood of Jesus.

Prayers against blood suckers and flesh eaters.

Covenant with blood suckers and flesh eaters, break over my life, waiting to manifest on my day of delivery, break in the name of Jesus Christ.

I command blood suckers and flesh eaters, to lose their power over my life.

Blood suckers and flesh eaters, walking around my environment, be arrested in the name of Jesus Christ.

Environmental altars of blood suckers and flesh eaters in my environment, be destroyed by fire in the name of Jesus Christ.

I withdraw my womb from the altar of blood suckers and flesh eaters in the name of Jesus Christ.

Every rage of blood suckers and flesh eaters against my baby, be dashed in the name of Jesus Christ.

Every curse that brought blood suckers and flesh eaters on my life, be broken by the power in the blood of Jesus Christ.

Evil agreement of blood suckers and flesh eaters over my life, in any hospital where my delivery will be taken, be cancelled by the power in the blood of Jesus.

I shut the door against the blood suckers and flesh eaters in my life in the name of Jesus Christ.

Every channel through which blood suckers and flesh eaters are using to gain entrance into my life, be destroyed in the name of Jesus Christ.

Praying for divine provision.

Covenant of poverty and lack in my marriage, that wants to manifest after I deliver my baby, break in the name of Jesus Christ.

Power of the devourer, roaring against my finances at the time of my pregnancy, be arrested in the name of Jesus Christ.

The head of my baby, refuse to cooperate with poverty in the name of Jesus Christ.

Doors of divine financial opportunities open for me and my family in the name of Jesus Christ.

O Lord, reveal to me, the hidden riches of secret places in the name of Jesus Christ.

I arrest and destroy every devourer on rampage against my finances in the name of Jesus Christ.

Foundational poverty and lack, break and release my family in the name of Jesus Christ.

Satanic bank, caging my money, be destroyed by fire and release my money in the name of Jesus Christ.

Evil dedication to family idol, sponsoring poverty in my life, break by the power in the blood of Jesus Christ.

Marine witchcraft covenant, caging my money, break by the power in the blood of Jesus Christ.

Spirit spouse, siphoning my money and my opportunities, I arrest you in the name of Jesus Christ.

I shall not nurse my baby with the garment of poverty in the name of Jesus Christ.

Every devourer hiding to swallow my money in the obstetric process, I bind you in the name of Jesus Christ.

Every spirit of ignorance, assigned to devour my money, during the obstetric process, be disgraced in the name of Jesus Christ.

Witchcraft embargo over my financial prosperity, break in the name of Jesus Christ.

Arrow of the wasters, programmed into the life of my unborn child, come out by fire in the name of Jesus Christ.

Destiny helpers, locate my destiny in the name of Jesus Christ.

As I deliver my baby, there shall be divine connection to people that matter, and kings and princes shall bless me in the name of Jesus Christ.

Environmental poverty, my life is not your candidate, release my money in the name of Jesus Christ.

Yoke of financial limitation, break and release me in the name of Jesus Christ.

Prayers for divine protection.

Every witchcraft meeting, gathered to destroy me or my unborn child, scatter by fire in the name of Jesus Christ.

Lay your hands on your Tommy, and pray, fire of the Holy Ghost, incubate the baby in my womb in the name of Jesus Christ.

I acquire the Immunity of the Holy Ghost against serpents and scorpions that want to attack me or my baby in the name of Jesus Christ.

I laminate my baby with the power in the blood of Jesus Christ.

Open doors to witchcraft attacks in my life and my unborn baby's life, be closed forever in the name of Jesus Christ.

Evil arrows, targeted against me and my baby, backfire in the name of Jesus Christ.

Witchcraft mirror, monitoring me and my unborn baby, break and scatter to pieces in the name of Jesus Christ.

Every wicked relative, using blood as a ladder to attack me and my unborn child, be exposed and be disgraced by fire in the name of Jesus Christ.

Power of satanic ritual and sacrifice, fashioned against me and my unborn baby, be rendered impotent in the name of Jesus Christ.

Owners of evil load prepared for me or my unborn baby, appear and carry your load in the name of Jesus Christ.

Evil medical report issued in the hospital, against me or my unborn child, catch fire and burn to ashes in the name of Jesus Christ.

Evil altars attacking me and my unborn child, be destroyed by fire in the name of Jesus Christ.

Evil pattern of miscarriage, break and release me and my baby in the name of Jesus Christ.

My baby, reject any congenital malformations in the name of Jesus Christ.

Angels of the living God, being to monitor and protect me and my pregnancy in the name of Jesus Christ.

I bear on my body the marks of the Lord Jesus, let no demon trouble me in the name of Jesus Christ.

I speak to every roaring lion on assignment against my baby and myself to devour us, be paralysed in the name of Jesus Christ.

Every witchcraft garment over my life, catch fire and burn to ashes in the name of Jesus Christ.

O Lord, expose and disgrace every witchcraft caterer in the market place, polluting my life and unborn child in the name of Jesus Christ.

Weapons of the enemy, against me and my unborn baby, perish by fire in the name of Jesus Christ.

Prayers against covenants fashioned against me and my baby.

Environmental covenants fashioned against me and my baby, break in the name of Jesus Christ.

Every evil covenant in my environment that I entered into through food, that is serving as a ladder for the enemy to enter my life break by the power on the blood of Jesus Christ.

Unconscious covenant that I have entered into in times past, through sex, that wants to attack me or my baby, be broken by the power in the blood of Jesus Christ.

Every witchcraft covenant in the life of my parents, that is manifesting against me or my unborn baby, be destroyed by the power in the blood of Jesus Christ.

Marine witchcraft covenant, break and release me and my unborn baby in the name of Jesus Christ.

Every unconscious covenant that I entered unto through consultation with the medium, be broken by the power in the blood of Jesus Christ.

Any foundational blood covenant, that blood suckers and flesh eaters want to use on the day of my delivery, break in the name of Jesus Christ.

Any covenant with my ex- boyfriend or girlfriend that wants to manifest against my wellbeing and that of my baby, break in the name of Jesus Christ.

Covenant with the earth, waiting to manifest against me on the day of my delivery, be cancelled by the power in the blood of Jesus Christ.

Evil covenant with the strongman of my in-law's house, break and release me in the name of Jesus Christ.

Evil covenant that I entered through laying of hands that wants to work against me or my unborn baby, break in the name of Jesus Christ.

Any evil covenant that I entered into through the use of other people's clothing, break in the name of Jesus Christ.

Every covenant that I entered into through my attendance in any evil festival, break and release me in the name of Jesus Christ.

Every unconscious evil covenant that I entered into on the day that I registered in the present hospital that I plan to put to bed, be exposed and be disgraced in the name of Jesus Christ.

Familiar spirit covenant with death on the day of my delivery, break in the name of Jesus Christ.

Demons that are joined with me in any evil covenant, scatter by the power in the blood of Jesus Christ.

Evil covenant on the day of my wedding that is waiting to manifest for affliction on the day of my delivery, break by the power in the blood of Jesus Christ.

I and my unborn baby refuse to be a victim of evil covenants in the name of Jesus Christ.

Occultic covenant fashioned against me and my unborn baby, break in the name of Jesus Christ.

Breaking curses fashioned against the joy of child birth.

Every foundational curse that is waiting to manifest on the day that I will put to bed, break by the power in the blood of Jesus Christ.

Any curse issued against my safe delivery by any witchcraft agent, break in the name of Jesus Christ.

Generational curse waiting to manifest against my health and that of my baby, break in the name of Jesus Christ.

Environmental curse crying against my life and that of my baby, break and release us in the name of Jesus Christ.

Any cursed midwife, that is programmed to commit an error on the day of my delivery, receive deliverance in the name of Jesus Christ.

Curses over the hospital that I registered to put to bed, be broken in the name of Jesus Christ.

Any curse issued by my mother in-law that wants to manifest against my joy of motherhood, be broken in the name of Jesus Christ.

Any evil altar, sponsoring evil pronouncements against my life, catch fire and be destroyed in the name of Jesus Christ.

Curse of sickness in my pregnancy and after childbirth, fashioned against me and my unborn baby, be broken in the name of Jesus Christ.

Curse of poverty, issued to manifest during my pregnancy and after childbirth, break on the name of Jesus Christ.

Curse of rejection, waiting to manifest against me and my unborn baby, break in the name of Jesus Christ.

Curse of shame and reproach, fashioned against me and my unborn baby, break in the name of Jesus Christ.

Curse of untimely death, sponsored by the kingdom of darkness against me and my unborn baby, before or after delivery, break in the name of Jesus Christ.

Curse of medical emergency and impossibility, during my labour, break in the name of Jesus Christ.

Curse of insanity, fashioned against me after childbirth, break in the name of Jesus Christ.

Curse of still birth, you shall not prosper in my life on the day of delivery in the name of Jesus Christ.

Every curse empowering flesh eaters and blood suckers over my life, break in the name of Jesus Christ.

By the power in the blood of Jesus Christ, I blot out any curse hiding in my life and waiting to manifest on the day of my delivery in the name of Jesus Christ.

Evil pronouncements against my glory, or the glory of my unborn baby, I break your power in the name of Jesus Christ.

Any demon, enforcing the curse of tragedy and disaster in my life, be rendered impotent in the name of Jesus Christ.

Prayers for an effective and safe delivery.

Times and seasons, I decree you shall not work against my wellbeing and that of my baby in the name of Jesus Christ.

You the earth, water and elements, you shall cooperate with me on the day of my delivery in the name of Jesus Christ.

Wisdom of God from above, descend and silence every demon that wants to rage on the day of my delivery in the name of Jesus Christ.

Anointing for easy delivery, fall upon my life in the name of Jesus Christ.

Every evil record, written against me on the day of delivery, I wipe you off by the power in the blood of Jesus Christ.

Wisdom from above, incubate the life of the doctors and nurses that will take my delivery on the appointed date in the name of Jesus Christ.

Any doctor or nurse that wants to cause complications on my day of delivery, angels of God, go forth and arrest them in the name of Jesus Christ.

My head (hold your head), you shall not be bewitched on the day of my delivery in the name of Jesus Christ.

The head if my baby, I decree you shall not be bewitched, you shall cooperate with the obstetric process.

Witchcraft agent assigned to torment my destiny on my day of delivery, you are liar, be frustrated in the name of Jesus Christ.

The head of my baby shall not refuse to cooperate with my passage on the day of delivery in the name of Jesus Christ.

Holy Spirit, lead me to make the right move at the right time in the name of Jesus Christ.

Everything that is meant to happen during my delivery shall happen at the right time, there shall be no hindrance, there shall be no delays in the name of Jesus Christ.

Any demon, any masquerade, any personality appearing to me in the dream, in order to hinder my safe delivery, judgement of God, fall upon them in the name of Jesus Christ.

Every evil altar, that will call my name for evil on the day of my delivery, or in my pregnancy, be destroyed by fire in the name of Jesus Christ.

On the day of my delivery, there shall not be failure of electricity, or water supply, everything shall work smoothly to the glory of God.

Satanic traffic that wants to delay me on the day of my delivery, clear away by fire in the name of Jesus Christ.

Evil voice assigned to mislead me on the day of my delivery, I silence you in the name of Jesus Christ.

Evil imaginations, manifesting against my safe delivery, and about the obstetric process, clear away by fire in the name of Jesus Christ.

My head, refuse to cooperate with witchcraft summon, in the name of Jesus Christ.

Breaking the yoke of evil dedication against me and my unborn child.

Every demon assigned to arrack me or my baby, during pregnancy and childbirth as a result of ancestral dedication, be arrested in the name of Jesus Christ.

Any soul-tie fashioned against me or my baby sponsoring evil dreams, break in the name of Jesus Christ.

Any equipment, in the hospital that I have registered, that wants to work against me, I break your power in the name of Jesus Christ.

Every dedication in my area that will likely work against the growth and wellbeing of my unborn baby, break in the name of Jesus Christ.

Evil dedication to the river, by my parents that wants to work against my safe delivery and the wellbeing of my baby, break in the name of Jesus Christ.

Evil dedication in the life of any nurse, doctor, or hospital staff, that may likely work contrary on the day of my delivery, break in the mighty name of Jesus Christ.

Ancestral dedication to familiar spirits, break and release me in the mighty name of Jesus Christ.

Any evil dedication of the midwife's labour couch, that wants to swallow the glory of my unborn child, be broken in the name of Jesus Christ.

Every witchcraft hand of the satanic doctor or midwife, that wants to dedicate my baby on my day of delivery, I break your power and command you to wither by fire in the name of Jesus Christ.

And evil power that wants to dedicate my unborn baby, as a result of a place that I entered or sat unknowingly, lose your grip in the name of Jesus Christ.

Any evil idol name that I am being called, that has dedicated my baby indirectly I break your power over the life of my baby in the mighty name of Jesus Christ.

Any covenant of evil dedication that I pushed myself or my unborn baby into as a result of any careless utterance or action, be broken in the mighty name of Jesus Christ.

Evil parental dedication to the occult, affecting my unborn baby negatively, break in the name of Jesus Christ.

I jump out of any witchcraft pot of evil dedication in the mighty name of Jesus Christ.

I break the power and authority of any demon that I have been unconsciously dedicated to that wants to affect the growth, development and wellbeing of my unborn baby in the name of Jesus Christ.

Evil dedication in my husband's family, assigned to bring shame and reproach against me and my baby, during pregnancy and childbirth, be broken in the name of Jesus Christ.

Every yoke of evil dedication working against me and my unborn child, break in the name of Jesus Christ.

Evil access to my life or my baby's life from any evil altar, I cut you off in the mighty name of Jesus Christ.

Any demon, that I was unconsciously dedicated to, that is appearing to me in the dream, your end has come, expire in the mighty name of Jesus Christ.

Any demon that is stealing from me or my unborn baby, because of any soul tie or evil dedication, I break your power and influence over my life in the mighty name of Jesus Christ.

Divine revelation

O Lord, show me the hospital, where you want me to deliver, and do not allow me to walk into witchcraft coven to deliver my baby.

O Lord, show me every person that you have ordained to be an angel unto me in my pregnancy and childbirth, in the name of Jesus Christ.

Every serpent and scorpion on assignment against my pregnancy and childbirth, be exposed and be disgraced in the mighty name of Jesus Christ.

Father Lord, show me the best procedure that will bring my baby to this world without any complications in the mighty name of Jesus Christ.

Father reveal to me, any food that I am eating, that is not good for my health and not in the best interest of my baby.

O Lord, show me whom the doctor that I have registered to deliver my baby is. Show me his spiritual identity in the name of Jesus Christ.

O Lord, show me the spiritual identity of all the staff in the hospital that I registered with to deliver my baby (mention the names of the staff, one-by-one), in the name of Jesus Christ.

Anyone in my family, hiding in the dark that attack me and my unborn baby, light of God, expose and disgrace such a person in the name of Jesus Christ.

O Lord, show me how to correct every anomaly against my pregnancy and childbirth, in the name of Jesus Christ.

Father Lord, show me every pit that the enemy has dug for me and my baby, in the mighty name of Jesus Christ.

O Lord, show me secrets about the life of my unborn child in the name of Jesus Christ.

Father Lord, show me the don'ts about the life of my baby, as you showed the parents of Jesus and Samson on the name of Jesus Christ.

Father Lord, show me the assignment you have for my unborn baby on earth, in the name of Jesus Christ.

Father reveal to me, prophetically, the name you would like to give to my baby, after he or she is born, that will bring forth your glory in the name of Jesus Christ.

O Lord, give me a child of prophecy in the name of Jesus Christ.

O Lord, give daily revelation concerning the life of my baby in the mighty name of Jesus Christ.

Father Lord, reveal to me every faulty foundation in my life, that will likely affect the health, growth and wellbeing of my unborn baby in the name of Jesus Christ.

Every ancestral demon on my husbands' side, attacking my pregnancy and childbirth, Holy spirit, expose and disgrace them in the name of Jesus Christ.

A table is given in Chapter 11 regarding how to use these prayer points. Note that your dreams should be recorded on a daily basis and given to your Pastor for interpretation, if he has the gift, or ability. He could also anoint with oil, or lay hands.

Our coaching and mentoring programs are available on abayomi.olugbemiga@gmail.com

CHAPTER 7

NUTRITION AND HYGIENE IN PREGNANCY

If you make certain mistakes, and you become vulnerable, when you shouldn't, then we could refer to that as self bewitchment. The Bible says, "my people perish for lack of knowledge" (Hosea 4:6). There are things that you need to know as a pregnant woman that will contribute to your health, the health of your baby, and ensure a safe delivery. A knowledge of nutrition, hygiene, exercise, complications in pregnancy, and signs to expect in labour are worth exploring.

Nutrition

Balanced diet. As a pregnant woman, it is pretty important not just to have access to all the necessary nutrients, but in the right proportions. If a particular nutrient is lacking in a person's diet consistently, then it leads to a deficiency disease. The temptation all over the world is for a pregnant woman to take junk foods, partly due to poverty, and partly due to ignorance. A diet that is not balanced in carbohydrates, proteins, fats and oils, vitamins, minerals, and trace elements will affect the health of the mother, and the health and development of the baby.

Folic acid, iron and calcium. Folic acid is an important constituent of the diet of a pregnant woman because it helps in the neural tube development. In early pregnancy if this is affected, the formation of the brain or spinal cord may be affected leading to spina bifida, anencephaly, and encephalocele which all have an effect on infant mortality rates.

Iron should be taken through dietary sources like green leaf vegetables, beef liver, legumes, nuts and seed etc. Iron supplements in form of tonics and capsules are good as well for good blood formation. Anaemia is a common problem in pregnant women that could lead to premature death, and low birth weight of the babies and post-partum depression in the mother. Calcium is responsible for good growth and development of the bones in the baby.

Limit intake of caffeine. Too much of caffeine in the diet of a pregnant woman can cause miscarriage, still birth, low birth weight, and low birth weight for gestational age. Drinks rich on caffeine include coffee, tea, soft drinks, and energy drinks.

Pregnant women should avoid alcohol totally, because of the Foetal Alcohol Spectrum Disorders (FASD). The first of these disorders is the foetal Alcohol Syndrome (FAS), which causes growth deficiencies, central nervous system dysfunction, development delays, and facial anomalies. The second is Alcohol Related Neurodevelopmental Disorder (ARND), which causes intellectual disabilities, problems with behaviour and learning. The third is Alcohol Related Birth Defects (ARBD) are birth defects as a result of alcohol consumption. The fourth is Neurobehavioral Disorder Associated with Prenatal Alcohol Exposure (ND-PAE) which causes behaviour disorders and learning disabilities.

In addition to these, alcohol can cause miscarriage, still birth, pre-term birth, and low birth weight.

Stay hydrated. As a pregnant woman, you need to stay hydrated, because water helps to maintain a good blood volume of blood and the amniotic fluid volume.

Special precautions. Foods that are not properly cooked can be dangerous for consumption by a pregnant woman, like seafood, eggs and meat. High mercury fish should be avoided because it has a negative effect on the baby's neurological and behavioural development.

Sugar and salt consumption should be reduced to the barest minimum. Excessive salt can lead to hypertension in the mother and affect the kidneys in the baby. Excessive salt in the body can cause retention of water in the body, and reduce water available to build the volume of the amniotic fluid, as well as affect its electrolyte balance. High intake of sugar may cause gestational diabetes, obesity or overweight, behavioural and cognitive problems.

Hygiene

Hand washing. The hands need to be washed before and after eating because of the risk of infections.

Skin care. Attention should be paid to the care of the skin, which should be washed daily and many times, using mild soap, and a moisturiser.

Oral hygiene. The teeth and mouth should be washed, and the teeth should be checked with the dentist when necessary. Research shows that infection in the gum can be transmitted through blood and affects the baby through the blood route. Furthermore, a link has been found between dental infections and the incidence of pre-eclampsia.

Clothes and underwear. These should not be dirty, and should be changed daily, especially the underwear. Dirty pants can harbour infections that stay around the vulva and can find its way to the womb, apart from the fact that it is uncomfortable.

Food hygiene. Don't eat indiscriminately, and every fruit and vegetables must be washed thoroughly before consumption, because they can carry bacteria or other viruses which could have an effect on the alimentary or respiratory system of the mother, and also the baby. Fish, meat, poultry, and eggs should be properly cooked.

Cups, plates and cutlery. These should not be shared with anyone, because of cross infection.

Clean the bathroom thoroughly and make it nice. The things there should be neatly kept and well arranged, and towels must be kept on the floor to absorb water that could cause a fall. The cleaning after using the toilet is use the wipe from the vulva towards the anus, to prevent infection.

Pets. Pregnant women should try as much as possible to avoid direct contact with pets because of the risk of transmission of infections. Cats could give toxoplasmosis, whilst birds and reptiles could transmit salmonella. Also avoid cleaning the litter of these pets, and train them not jump on you. Wash your hands thoroughly each time you handle pets, and make sure they take their immunisations as well as deworm them. Do not allow the plates and eating utensils of pets to mix up with yours.

Environmental hygiene. Ensure there is cross ventilation and adequate ventilation. Beddings and towels should be washed weekly or periodically.

Public spaces. Avoid close contact with the crowd, because you never can know who has an infection. Use hand sanitizers and wipes, making sure to take every vaccination due.

CHAPTER 8

COMPLICATIONS IN PREGNANCY

There are certain complications in pregnancy that a pregnant woman needs. To be able to detect, in order to act appropriately, and promptly, or to note it should in case it happens to then or other people in the future.

These are:

Gestational diabetes mellitus (GDM) is when the blood sugar in a pregnant woman is excessive. This comes with a tendency to pre-eclampsia, and pregnancy induced high blood pressure, prolapsed umbilical cord, placental abruption, miscarriage, premature labour, or still birth. On occasions, this condition may need high risk pregnancy care. If left untreated, it can cause serious problems for the mother and unborn child. In most mothers with gestational diabetes, labour has to be induced between the 35th and 40th week of pregnancy, if the diabetes is not controlled. There is a possibility for a caesarean section if the baby becomes too big. There is a likelihood of foetal death if the case is not handled properly.

Pre-eclampsia. This is usually characterised by a high blood pressure and presence of excess proteins in urine, during pregnancy. The symptoms of this condition include a high blood pressure, excess protein in the urine, headaches that do not get relief after using common pain killers, abdominal pains, nausea and vomiting, breathlessness, changes in vision, and decreased urine output. Swelling of the feet in pregnancy is common, and to some extent can be normal. However, swelling, especially in the face, and hands are deviations from normal and suspicion of pre-eclampsia is relevant. One beneficial approach to the prevention of eclampsia is to regularly monitor, and check blood pressure and urine, during ante-natal checks. Another thing is to eat healthy and do exercises as appropriate. Treatment of any underlying medical conditions is necessary. In the treatment of mild pre-eclampsia, monitoring is necessary, good rest is essential.

In severe cases of eclampsia, hospitalisation is necessary. Medications not just directed towards monitoring blood pressure, but to aid breathing of the baby, and prevent seizures in the mother, which is a possibility. An ultimate solution to severe pre-eclampsia, is the delivery of the baby, and this decision is based upon the severity of the condition, and gestational age.

Pre-term Labour. This means labour that begins before 37 weeks of pregnancy. When there is pre-term labour, which is not well taken care of, it leads to pre-term labour. Pre-term babies face several challenges, including respiratory problems, difficulties in feeding, and developmental delays.

Which factors increase the risk of pre-term labour? The first factor is that if there is a history of pre-term labour, or pre-term births in previous pregnancies. Secondly, when there is a multiple pregnancy, in which case the ultrasound scan has revealed that a mother is carrying twins or triplets, they need to be very careful. Third one is uterine or cervical abnormalities, e.g. short cervix or abnormalities of the uterus. For example, a woman that has a lot of scar tissue in the womb due to several evacuations, could be a candidate of pre-term birth. Infections of the amniotic fluid, lower genital tract, or urinary tract could also affect the baby and cause pre-term birth. Microorganisms release cytokines and prostaglandins in excess, and can induce uterine contractions.

The fifth factor is chronic conditions. This includes high blood pressure, diabetes mellitus, and auto-immune disorders. High blood pressure and diabetes mellitus have been linked to pre-term labour in many ways. Any mother having any of these should report to the doctor urgently. Sixth factor is your lifestyle! Do you take alcohol, do you smoke or take illicit drugs? Seventh thing to note is that high levels of stress also lead to pre-term birth, especially if it is of an extended time. A pregnant woman should try and avoid all forms of physical and emotional stress; however, the case may be.

The eighth factor to note is that placental problems may present e.g. placental abruption. Placental abruption is when the placenta separates from the inner wall of the uterus before birth. The main noticeable symptom is bleeding from the vagina. Other symptoms are abdominal pain, back pain, and abdominal contractions. The second placental problem is placenta previa which is usually noticed after 20 weeks of pregnancy after an ultrasound scan. This is a situation whereby the placenta is formed every close to the neck of the uterus, and blocks it partially or completely. The signs of placenta previa include a bright red haemorrhage, without pain, and possibly with contractions. Majority of the partial or complete placenta previa resolve before delivery.

The ninth complication during pregnancy that I will like to mention here is vaginal bleeding. Vaginally bleeding may be noticed when there is ectopic pregnancy, spontaneous abortion, placenta previa, placental abruption, preterm labour, and molar pregnancy. Amniotic fluid abnormalities may also cause a problem. The tenth case, includes abnormalities of the amniotic fluid. The first is of these anomalies is Oligohydramnios means very little amniotic fluid, and is caused by drugs, utero-placental insufficiency, ruptured membranes and foetal abnormalities. It is characterised by leaking of the amniotic fluid, low amniotic fluid on ultrasound, retarded growth, low maternal weight gain, abdominal discomfort, and sudden drop in foetal heart rate.

The other amniotic fluid abnormality is polyhydramnios. This is when the amniotic fluid is in excess, and is caused by gestational diabetes, multiple pregnancy, infections of the foetus, disturbed foetal swallowing, and genetic disorders of the baby. The signs are sensations of tightness in the upper stomach, cramplings or contractions, shortness of breath, heartburn, difficulty pooing, peeing more often, swelling in the vulva, legs and feet, and urinary tract infections.

CHAPTER 9

FAITH IN PREGNANCY.

"Faith is the substance of things hoped for, and the evidence of things not seen." (Hebrews 11:1). However, faith is believing that something is bound to happen, but something must accompany that belief. In James 2:17 the bible says, "even so, faith, if it hath not works, is dead." We need to substantiate our faith by our works, to make faith come alive.

Faith is absolute confidence in the word of God, and unshaken trust in the power of God to save and to deliver. Irrespective of how tough things may seem, someone who has faith is never afraid, intimidated, or neither is he/she stoppable.

There are two scriptures that are relevant, and that we need to concentrate upon:

Isaiah 66:9

Do I bring to the moment of birth, and not give delivery?" says the Lord. "Do I close up the womb when I bring to delivery?"

John 16:21

A woman giving birth to a child has pain because her time has come; but when her baby is born, she forgets the anguish because of her joy that a child is born into the world.

What are the desires of a pregnant woman, and what are the expectations?

1. Protection for her and the baby in the time of pregnancy and afterwards
2. Immunity to diseases, and good health during pregnancy
3. Delivery of a healthy, and well-formed baby
4. Safe delivery of the baby without loss of blood or trauma
5. That God should preserve her life at the time of child delivery and after.

6. Prayers for the staff involved in antenatal, perinatal, and postnatal care.

Desire and faith go hand in hand for a Christian. When you have a desire, you pray, and God reveals his word, concerning that which you have asked. The absolute confidence in the word you have received from the Lord, as you believe and behave it gives birth to your earnest desires. Performance added to faith is miracles. Keep adding works to faith as you prevent self-bewitchment as shown in the earlier chapter of this book.

How do you achieve your desires by faith as a pregnant mother?

1. *Surrender your life to Christ.* Jesus says, "I am the way, the truth, and the life." (John 14:6). Once you surrender the steering wheel of your life to Jesus, and allow him to drive, he will always drive you to the shores of fulfilment and joy. He says come unto me, all ye that labour and are heavy laden, and I will give you rest (Matthew 11:28). If you haven't

confessed Jesus as your Lord and saviour, say this:

Father, I make you Lord and saviour over my life, I forsake the devil and all his evil works. Thank you, Lord Jesus.

2. *Repent from sin.* The Bible says in James 4:17, that "to him that knoweth to do good and doeth it not, it is sin." By virtue of God's word and commands, there are things you ought to do. Failure to do any or all of them is sin! Sins in your mind, like pride, hatred, unforgiveness, malice, envy, covetousness, arrogance, and the likes, are all not acceptable. As a pregnant woman, for you to experience healing and great peace, for example, you need to forgive your in-laws, your neighbours, and any errant co-workers. This is when you can actually concentrate and focus unhindered, to get what you are believing God for. Also watch the sins of words, in evil speaking, negative speaking, and others. The actions too must be watched to conform to God's will. Each time you want to do something, ask yourself, "is God happy with what I want to do"? In 1

Corinthians 10:31, it says, "whether therefore ye eat or drink, or whatsoever ye do, do all to the glory of God." Eating what you are not supposed to eat in pregnancy is sin and dangerous!

3. *Study and meditation of God's word.* The word of God is the direction he expects you to go, and your life finds direction with the word of God, when propelled by faith, especially violently. As you meditate in God's word, chapter by chapter, you discover hidden secrets for unlimited success. It is worthwhile to study a chapter of the bible, daily. The Psalms, Ecclesiastes, Proverbs, and the New Testament are especially helpful. As you continue to study, your spirit is ignited, and you have revelations and dreams to guide and protect you in pregnancy. God's power is activated with revelation and faith. Part of demonstration of your faith is walking in righteousness and holiness.

4. *Fervent prayers.* Prayer is communication with God, and has to be fervent, (James 5:16) that is felt strongly in your spirit. There should be no distractions, as the prayer time should be

a quiet time. Psalm 4:4 describes, "a posture for prayer stand in awe and sin not, commune with your own heart on your bed and be still." Mind you, when you pray and be still, allow a thought to drop in your spirit. This is the spirit's response to your prayers, if it is in alignment with the word of God. Pray, without doubt, and as you believe, the word of God says you will receive. There are prayer strategies that have been highlighted under an earlier chapter in this book that are useful for you, to exercise your spirit and to receive great things from God.

5. *Write your dreams and revelations.* When you study the word, and pray to God, you will have a multitude of revelations, which is God's plan, purpose, and intentions for your life. The word of God is the truth and incorruptible, and this is what you should believe and allow to create a foundation for every thought, word, attitude and action. You could enrol on our mentorship or coaching program.

6. *Deal with negativity.* The Bible says in 2 Corinthians 10:5, "Casting down

imaginations and every high thing that exalts itself against the knowledge of God, and bringing into captivity, every **thought** to the obedience of Christ." Mark 11:23 says, "For verily I say unto you, that whosoever shall say unto this mountain, be thou removed and be cast into the sea; and shall **not doubt** in his heart, but **shall believe** that those things which he saith shall come to pass; he shall whatsoever he saith." Two other things that constitute negativity are your emotions and your feelings. In all, at all times, a pregnant woman should deal with negative imaginations, thoughts, feelings, emotions, doubt and unbelief when you are alone at home, or in the hours of the night, that may come against our safe delivery. The devil will bring different types of imaginations about your pregnancy and day of delivery, and if it is scary and you are afraid, you have agreed in principle. That fear could lead to a high blood pressure or make you prone to pre-eclampsia.

7. *Be positive minded.* The Bible makes us to know in Philippians 4:8, "whatsoever things

are true, whatsoever things are honest, whatsoever things are pure, whatsoever things are just, whatsoever things are lovely, and whatsoever things that are of a good report, if there be any virtue, and if there be any praise, think on these things." Whatsoever we think about should be positive things, and we should always imagine the best situations concerning out lives.

8. *Great expectations.* Everyone that ever received something great in the bible had great expectations continually. With faith is expectation, and with expectation is manifestation. When you go to see the nurses and doctors, do not fear, but have great expectations, as you buy things and shop for your baby things, have great expectations, and concerning the date of delivery, have great expectations.

9. *Word affirmations.* Lay your hands on your abdomen, and make confessions of the word of God positively, and severally, strengthens the spirit. For example, Isaiah 66:9 says, "Thank you Lord, because you shall bring me to the moment of birth O Lord, and give me

delivery." Isaiah 40:10 says, "I shall not fear O Lord, for you are with me." I refused to be dismayed because you are God. Isaiah 50:7 says, "For the Lord God will help me, therefore shall I not be confounded; therefore, I have set my face like a flint, and I know that I shall not be ashamed in the name of Jesus Christ."

10. *Add works to faith.* There are so many activities that fall under this, as faith without works is dead. The things we need to do from the human perspective, after God has released his word, are the amen to our prayers. They allow it to happen. Going to the hospital for antenatal care, and adhering to all instructions fall under this. Blessing people that take care of you is not out of place, as you are led. Fervent prayers are hard work as well. Whatever the case may be, substantiate your faith.

11. *Anointing with oil.* Have a bottle of olive oil, and your Pastor can pray in it, as you pray in it as well. Command the fire of God to incubate it, and command it to turn to the blood of Jesus. Decree it shall be for signs

and wonders, and that the power of resurrection of our Lord Jesus should enter into it. A handkerchief can also be prayed upon and you keep it with you, and for example, you could put it on your head, and command that the Holy spirit should fill you up in the name of Jesus Christ.

12. *Laying of hands.* Let men and women of God indeed lay hands on your shoulders, and pray for you. Each time a decree is made, laying hands on you, it transfers virtues and power. When you have a dream that is not pleasant, you could lay your hands and reverse the work of the enemy. It is also worthy to lay your hands on your abdomen and plant good things upon the life of your baby.

Chapter 10

SIGNS OF LABOUR AND STAGES OF LABOUR.

The first stage of labour – latent phase

It is good for a pregnant and expectant mother to understand the signs of labour, and the stages of labour. When there is an understanding, it is very easy to follow up. The Bible establishes the fact that every woman experiences labour pains, but that it will be over soon.

> *John 16:21*
>
> *"Woman giving birth to a child has pain because her time has come; but when her baby is born, she forgets the anguish, because of her joy that a child is born into the world."*

Labour is the process by which the baby and the placenta leave from the womb of the mother into the world. This occurs anything between the 37th to 42nd week. Anything before this is termed a pre-term birth.

It is worthy to mention that there is false labour are caused by Braxton Hicks contractions, and are usually felt within the second and third trimesters of labour. In false labour, the contraction frequency is low, usually once in 5-30 minutes, the intensity and strength of the contractions are weak, there is no decent, there is no dilation of the cervix, and there is no thinning or softening of the cervix, which are all present in the contractions as a result of true labour. The false labour pain is relieved by changes in position or walking from one place to the other.

The signs of labour are variable from person to person, but the initial one is that there is low back pain and usually the baby is resting the back of the head on the sacrum of the mother, whereby constipation too may result. There are also contractions or tightening that are felt in the uterus which initially are short and with considerable intervals, usually between 5 minutes to 30 minutes.

The intensity and cycles per minute increases as labour progress and the mother may discover there is a show.

A show is when the mucoid seal at the opening of the cervix is displaced and actually starts coming off.

This shows that the cervix is starting to open, soften and thin. The baby is getting ready to come to the world. This is then followed by breaking of the water. When there is breaking of the water, it means that the chorion and amniotic membranes are broken, giving way to escape of the amniotic fluid. This fluid provides a cushion for protection of the baby while in the womb and minimises the risks of infection.

The contractions are now increased in frequency and intensity, and this shows that labour is established. The pregnant woman should be in the hospital in this active phase, where everything suddenly changes, starting from the frequency and intensity of contractions. The countenance of the pregnant woman changes and oxytocin, or epidural anaesthesia is sometimes applied.

It is very essential for a mother to note that God already arranged everything to be easy for you, and you have to have faith in this. What is just happening is that the baby is trying to open the door to come out into the world, because it is time. This is why the show (mucoid plug comes off, and the membranes are broken. After this the conditions are faster as the baby is just simply insinuating that I have opened the door, I want to come out. Give way! Are you giving way or you are stressed and tensed, blocking the way?

The second stage of labour – delivery.

As the contractions are now increased, the cervix thins and softens with maximal dilation (10cm), and not less, because it is risky. When there is a descent, the midwives need to manage pain thereby making expulsion of the baby easy.

The midwives and the doctors try to administer relaxants, but care must be taken to administer it carefully, and slowly only at the peak of the contractions and that the baby is not sedated or becomes inactive. This could have terrible effects on the respiratory system of the baby, or cause a crash in the mother's blood pressure. Excess of relaxants might cause impaired ability of the mother to push, or altered mental status leading to confusion, depression, or dizziness. It may also cause abnormal heart patterns or foetal distress.

The baby may take several positions, known as presentations, but as the head of the baby descends into the pelvis, the shape of the pelvis tends to rotate the head of the baby.

There are also about a dozen positions or more that the midwives tell the mother to adopt during delivery. Sometimes, the mother kneels down prone on all four, while the midwife does some manoeuvre to the low back, and this is especially true when the occipital part of the baby's head is pressing too hard on the sacrum of the mother.

When every method to achieve a correct position of the head of the baby has failed, then they resolve to a caesarean section. Generally, the indications for a Caesarean section include:

Previous caesarean section delivery

Breech presentation

Dystopia

Foetal distress

Heart or brain condition of the mother

Placenta previa

A very small pelvis

High blood pressure of the mother

The third stage of labour.

The third stage of labour begins after the expulsion of the uterus, and ends with the expulsion of the placenta, usually less than an hour after the baby is delivered. If the process lasts for more than one hour, then the mother should be assessed for retention of the placenta.

Immediately the baby is delivered, the midwife waits until the cord stops pulsating, and this ensures that everything is okay and the baby is not at risk for anaemia. The cord is ligated and cut about 2cm - 5cm from the baby's belly, and the blood cleaned properly.

The mother after delivery may clutch to the baby, wrapped in a clean clothing, and after the breast is cleaned, socks from the mother. Right after birth, there are still contractions of the uterus, which helps to gradually help to separate the placenta from the uterus, as well as the membranes.

At this stage, many women bleed and the cause of unusual bleeding must be verified and taken care of. There should be minimal bleeding from the placenta. Post parturition haemorrhage is a common cause of maternal morbidity and mortality especially in developing countries. Post partum bleeding is usually controlled using 10 IU of oxytocin, especially in low income countries. Other remedies include, ergometrine, syntometrine, misoprostol, carboprost tromethamine, and carbetocin.

It is wise to tell the mother to urinate, to make sure the full bladder is not obstructing the placenta. A gentle cough may also prove useful in generating pressure to expel the placenta. The placenta may be expelled spontaneously or traction applied on the umbilical cord, with one hand while the other hand is used to monitor and hold the fundus of the uterus to prevent uterine inversion. A gentle pull within one hour with massaging of the uterus should expel the uterus. At the moment that the placenta is separated from the uterine wall, there is a gush of blood, the placenta could be felt at the lower abdomen, the cord outside the vagina lengthens, the membranes and placenta can be seen visibly in between the labia.

If the placenta does not come out with the above, the woman should be examined for a retained placenta. Antibiotics should be administered. Depending on the assessment, general or regional anaesthesia could be employed through the spinal or epidural routes. Medications for relaxation and relief from pain like diazepam, ketamine, or midazolam could be administered intravenously.

Once the placenta is expelled or removed, the cotyledons of the placenta should be checked if they are complete. The blood pressure, arterial pulse or body temperature should be checked every 15 minutes for one hour, and 30 minutes intervals thereafter., to make sure there is no serious loss of blood, which could prove fatal.

Fourth stage of labour.

This stage starts immediately after the placenta is expelled, until the mother stabilises clinically. There are measurements that need to be taken in this process, before the mother and the baby are transferred to the post-natal ward.

The baby is allowed to suck the mother's breast, and this helps contraction of the uterus, release of endogenous oxytocin, and helps to control post partum haemorrhage. Vital signs that are observed at this stage.

Tears or lacerations of the perineum, as well as episiotomy sites need to be neatly and appropriately sutured. The genital tract needs to be examined for bleeding, especially coming from the vaginal orifice, periodically.

The fundus of the uterus is massaged to stimulate contraction and reduce the risk of post-partum haemorrhage, expel blood clots, and monitor uterine tone and size. The midwife should make sure that the womb is completely evacuated of placental tissue, and perhaps a hiding foetus!

The weight of the baby, the head circumference, abdomen circumference, chest circumference, length of umbilical cord, patency of orifices like the mouth, ears, genitalia, anus and nostrils need to be checked. The spine also needs to be thoroughly checked.

It is worthy to note that the midwife needs to check the respiratory rate (40-60 b/min), heart rate (122-140 b/min), motor activity, skin colour, temperature (35.5°C – 37°C), bladder and bowel activities.

CHAPTER 11

AN OVERVIEW OF THE DELIVERANCE OF THE FOETUS.

The bible (Ephesians 6:12) makes us to know that we wrestle not against flesh and blood, but against principalities, powers, the rulers of darkness of this world, and spiritual wickedness in high places, and the pregnant woman is not left out in this battle with unseen spirits. Every pregnant woman should watch and be prepared to war in prayer against spiritual entities, whenever the need arises. Deliverance of the foetus is very wide, and should involve physical, medical, or scientific activities.

Observation is key in this case as the pregnant mother should watch out for signs of satanic attack against the pregnancy as highlighted in Chapter 4 of this book. As soon as any foul play is noticed like abnormal hearing, abnormal voice, abnormal visions, and any strange observations, physically or in the dream, a pregnant mother should tell the husband (if any) or phone a doctor, and they should report to the Pastor, or prayer warrior who would take the necessary action, spiritually.

Deliverance could take many forms, including counselling, praise and worship songs or even the confession of God's word. The pregnant sister and the husband should not rely only on the efforts of the prayer warriors alone, but trusted members of the husband's groups, or the wife's groups should also be aware of any spiritual needs of the family. Members of the wife's family that need to be aware are also informed to join in prayers or other support, like encouraging or preparing food. It is also good for the Pastor or his representatives to delegate people, especially from the house fellowship centre, or prayer warrior to liaise with the husband for visits and follow-up.

There should be laying of hands and anointing with oil. The pregnant woman also be taught how to anoint herself or how to learn the scriptures, all in an effort to instil faith in the mother.

One of the deliverance secrets is that God should reveal to a couple, the activities that are waiting them on the day of delivery. It is also good to know the various complications associated with pregnancy. All these are discussed in detail in this book.

Adding works to faith is essential, and the mother should be taught in the hospital, exercising that she could engage in safely. Exercises should not be tried without prescription, and sometimes, exercise testing may be carried out, before exercise prescription. It is important to eat a balanced diet, that is rich in fruits and vegetables. The ante-natal class should not be missed at any time, and questions should be asked where an issue is not clear. When the time of delivery is near, the pregnant mother should be familiar with the signs of labour, especially at the latent phase.

She should also be able to differentiate between true and false labour, all of which are explained clearly in this book.

The activities of the different stages of pregnancy should be known to the mother, so that she can follow actively during delivery especially for preventing or stopping haemorrhage. Post-partum haemorrhage is one of the leading causes of maternal morbidity and mortality worldwide, and should not be taken lightly.

A pregnant woman should read widely as regards to faith and what faith can do. Pregnant women should be taught thoroughly about faith and there is no better time to teach faith.

With adequate preparation and a sound knowledge of problems that could be encountered, there's no problem.

Deliverance Program.

A timetable has been suggested for the deliverance program for pregnant women. It should involve a fast starting from 8am to 12 noon, for a week in the month. The prayers are to be prayed every day, apart from one week in the month, where fasting is required. The fast is not mandatorily expected to be broken by 12 noon, as the candidate could break at any time if it is not convenient, or not fast at all, if the body system cannot cope with it.

Praise and worship, as well as forgiveness and mercy under Chapter 6 (Prayer Strategies for the Expectant Mother), are very important, and should be said daily. All other prayers are to be said are outlined under the same chapter, and should be prayed as shown below.

DELIVERANCE TIMETABLE

	8-9am	9-10am	10-11am	11-12am
Mon	1/2	3	4	8
Tue	1/2	6	9	4
Wed	1/2	6	5	7
Thu	1/2	8	7	5
Fri	1/2	9	3	4

Keys

1 – Praise and worship

2 - Forgiveness and mercy

3 – Prayers against flesh eaters and blood suckers

4 – Prayers for divine protection

5 – Prayers for divine provision

6 – Prayers against covenants fashioned against me and my baby

7 – Prayers for safe delivery

8 – Breaking the yoke of evil dedication against me and my unborn child

9 – Prayers for divine revelation

Printed in Great Britain
by Amazon